The Ultimate Keto Dinner Cookbook

50 Fast and Tasty Recipes to Burn fat and Stay Fit for Women Over 50

Katie Attanasio

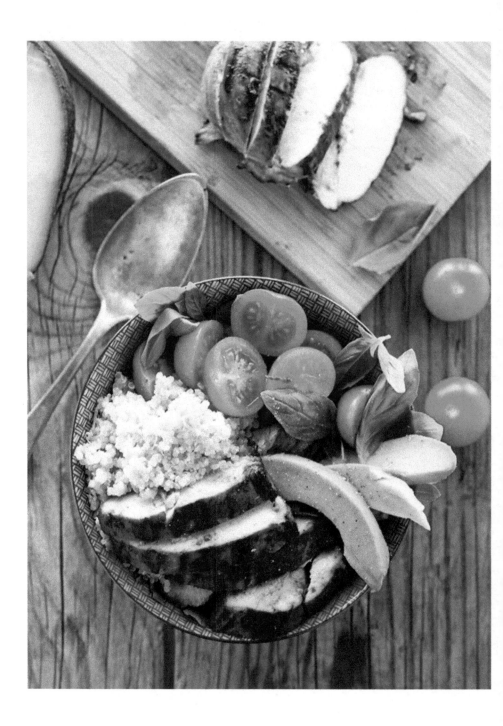

Table of Contents

50 Essential Dinner Recipes

1   No Bean Keto Chili In The Instant Pot

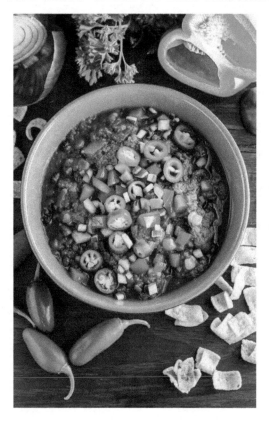

Servings: 6 | **Time**: 35 mins | **Difficulty**: Easy

Nutrients per serving: Calories: 222 kcal | Fat: 12.7g | Carbohydrates: 11.5g | Protein: 16.8g | Fiber: 3.3g

Ingredients

1/2 cup Onion, diced

1 1/2 Tbsp Olive oil, divided

1/2 Cup Celery sliced

1 Red pepper, diced

1 Tbsp Garlic, minced

4 tsp Chile powder

1 Lb Grass-fed 85% lean Ground beef

1 Tbsp Smoked Paprika

1/8 tsp Ground Allspice

1/4 tsp Cayenne pepper

1 Can Crushed tomatoes (14 oz)

1/2 Cup Water

1 Can Fire-roasted minced tomatoes (14oz)

2 Tbsp Tomato paste

Pinch of pepper

1 tsp Sea salt

1/4 cup Parsley chopped

2 Bay leaves

Method

1.   In the Instant Kettle, place 1/2 Tablespoon of the oil & switch to sauté mode. When it's hot, sauté the pepper, onion, celery & garlic for around 3 mins before they start to soften.

2.   Put the remaining oil and the beef & cook for around 3 to 4 mins, till it starts to turn brown. Drain out the extra fat.

3.   Put the paprika, chili powder, cayenne, then allspice, & simmer for 3 to 4 mins till the beef is entirely brown & no longer pink.

4.   Except for the Parsley, combine all the leftover ingredients & stir till well mixed. Cover your Instant Pot (please ensure it is sealed) & switch it to manual mode (high pressure should be adjusted instantly) & set it for ten min. Allow it to release steam naturally when cooked.

5.   Remove the cover and switch it to sauté mode when the steam is released. Cook, constantly stirring, for 2 to 4 mins, till some of the water has evaporated.

6.   Mix it in the Parsley & enjoy it.

2   Keto Shrimp Courgette Boats On The Grill

Servings: 4 | **Time**: 30 mins | **Difficulty**: Easy

Nutrients per serving: Calories: 180 kcal | Fat: 7.5g | Carbohydrates: 13.8g | Protein: 17g | Fiber: 4.1g

Ingredients

For The Courgette:

Two Large Courgette Squashes

1 Tsp Olive Oil

1/4 Tsp Salt

1/4 Tsp Ground Cayenne Pepper

For The Cauliflower Rice Salad:

One Small Onion, Roughly Chopped, Around

2 Cups One Large Bunch Of Asparagus

1 Tbsp Olive Oil, Plus 1 Tsp, Divided

1 Tsp Garlic, Chopped

Salt & Pepper

3 Tbsp Fresh Juice Of Lemon

3 Tbsp Fresh Basil, Chopped

2 Cups Cauliflower Florets, Cut Into Bite-Sized Pieces

For The Shrimp:

1 Tsp Olive Oil

1/2 Tsp Ground Cayenne Pepper

Lemon Zest, For Garnish

1 Tsp Honey

1/2 Pound Fresh Shrimp, Peeled & Deveined

Method

1.   Put the BBQ on a grill basket & preheat for around ten min on high heat.

2.   Slice the courgette lengthwise in half & scoop out a few of the inside, creating a boat. As the courgette softens when grilled, make sure to leave several along the edges. Use the olive oil to brush the courgette and sprinkle with cayenne pepper & salt.

3.   Toss the minced Onion and Asparagus only with oil & garlic in a wide bowl, then season with pepper & salt.

4.   Reduce the heat to med-high on the grill & put the Onion & Asparagus in the grill basket. Also, put the courgette directly on the grill, slice-side-down. Fry the vegetables for around ten min, till gently charred & excellent grill marks are created. Turn halfway through the courgette and stir the vegetables around. Remove & cover the vegetables from the grill & put them aside till ready for usage.

5.   Put the cauliflower in a big food processor as the vegetables cook & process till it falls into what appears like rice. Put in a wide bowl & microwave till soft, for 5-6 mins. If you like, you can steam the cauliflower in the oven as well.

6.   Put the barbecue heat back up to full again. Toss the oil, pepper, salt &honey with the shrimp, ensuring that the spices are spread equally. Put them on the grill & cook for around five min, till they are opaque & gently charred. Flip through halfway.

To Serve:

1.   Chop the onion as well as the grilled asparagus and put them into the cauliflower rice. Mix the leftover one tablespoon of olive oil, lemon juice & Basil together. Sprinkle with salt to taste.

2.   Scoop the mixture of cauliflower into the courgettes, really pack it in as far as you can, & add the shrimp on top. Add fresh lemon zest to garnish it.

3.   Now enjoy it.

3   Keto Sloppy Joes

Servings: 2 | **Time:** 5 mins | **Difficulty**: Easy

Nutrients per serving: Calories: 276 kcal | Fat: 18.8g | Carbohydrates: 4.4g | Protein: 23.2g | Fiber: 0.9g

Ingredients

1/2 tbsp Olive Oil

1 pound Ground Beef, (85%)

1/3 cup Green Onions, thinly sliced

3/4 cup Tomato Sauce (canned)

1 1/2 tbsp Tomato Paste

1/2 cup Low-Sodium Beef Broth

1 tbsp Monkfruit Sweetener

1 tbsp Worcestershire Sauce

1 tsp Red Wine Vinegar

1 tsp Chili Powder

1/2 tsp Sea Salt

1/2 tsp Prepared Yellow Mustard

pinch of Black Pepper

Lettuce, for serving

pinch of Crushed Red Pepper Flakes

Method

1.   Heat the olive oil in the big frying pan over med-high. Place the green onions & boil for a minute.

2.   Place the ground beef & cook for around five min till the beef is no different pink.

3.   In the bowl, mix all the rest of the ingredients up to Parsley. Place into the cooked beef & carry to a simmer.

4.   Decrease the heat to med after boiling & simmer till the sauce is thickened, around 9 to 10 mins.

5.   Spoon the combination over the lettuce & fill it with cheese & Parsley if necessary.

6.   Enjoy it.

4   Keto Steak With Garlic Butter Mushrooms

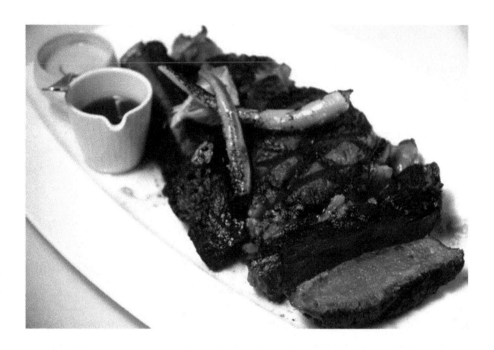

Servings: 4 | **Time**: 25 mins | **Difficulty:** Easy

Nutrients per serving: Calories: 292 kcal | Fat: 21.7g | Carbohydrates: 1.1g | Protein: 23.5g | Fiber: 0.4g

Ingredients

4 tsp Ghee, softened to room temperature

Sea salt

1 tsp Fresh garlic, chopped

1 Lb Grass-fed Top Sirloin Steak

For The Mushrooms:

2 Cups thinly sliced White mushrooms

2 tsp melted ghee

Sea salt

1 tsp minced fresh garlic

Method

1.   Preheat the barbecue to high heat

2.   With the paper towel, pat the steak off. Mix the ghee & garlic in the small bowl & scatter half of it on one steak side. Drizzle salt on it.

3.   Put the steak on it once the grill is hot, butter the side down & cook for 4 to 5 mins, till charred. Rub ghee combination on the top side, turn & cook till done-ness is desired. Take it from the heat, cover & leave to rest when cooking the mushrooms.

4.   In a cup, Add the melted ghee, mushrooms, garlic, and a splash of salt. Put two layers of tin foil over the top of each other & put the mushrooms in one layer in the middle. To make a packet, cover the sides up firmly.

5.   On the barbecue, put the mushrooms to fold a packet face up & grill for five min. Another 4 to 5 mins, or till the mushrooms are soft.

6.   Serve your mushrooms on the steak & enjoy it.

5   Keto Beef And Broccoli

Servings: 2 | **Time:** 1 hr 25 mins | **Difficulty:** Easy

Nutrients per serving: Calories: 344 kcal | Fat: 20.4g | Carbohydrates: 11.9g | Protein: 26.7g | Fiber: 3.3g

Ingredients

1 tsp minced & divided Fresh ginger

1/4 Cup Coconut aminos, divided

1 tsp minced & divided Fresh garlic

1 1/2 Tbsp Avocado oil, divided

8 Oz Flank steak, thinly sliced against the grain

1/4 Cup Reduced-sodium beef broth

2 1/2 Cups Broccoli, cut into big florets

Salt

1/2 tsp Sesame oil Sesame seeds for garnish

Green onion for garnish

Fried cauliflower rice

Method

1.   In a tiny bowl, mix 1 Tablespoon of the amino coconut, 1/2 Teaspoon of Garlic & ginger. Put & mix your beef into the marinade. For at least 1hr, cover & refrigerate.

2.   Heat 1 Tablespoon of oil over med heat in a big saucepan. Put the broccoli & cook for around 3 to 4 mins, constantly stirring, till it just starts to soften. Put the remaining garlic & ginger into the mixture and cook for 1 min.

3.   Lower the heat, cover the pan & cook for around 4-5 mins, till the broccoli is soft and crisp. Occasionally, stir it.

4.   Move the broccoli to the plate when cooked. Turn the heat to med/high & put the leftover 1/2 Tablespoon of oil to it. Put the marinated beef & cook for around 2 to 3 mins, till golden brown. Stir back the broccoli in.

5.   Mix the remaining amino coconut, sesame oil & broth in a shallow bowl. Place it into the skillet & simmer till it is only starting to thicken, stirring continuously for around 1-2 min—season with salt.

6.   Serve with sesame seeds & green onion on cauliflower rice.

6   Keto Philly Cheesesteak With Cauliflower & Stuffed Peppers

Servings: 6 | **Time:** 50 mins | **Difficulty**: Easy

Nutrients per serving: Calories: 379 kcal | Fat: 22.9g | Carbohydrates: 11g | Protein: 32.7g | Fiber: 2.3g

Ingredients

For the Onions:

1 Tbsp Olive oil Salt

Two big onions sliced around 1/2 thick

For the Peppers:

Six tiny Green bell peppers

1 Lb Beef top sirloin steak

1 Tbsp Olive oil

Salt

2 cups Cauliflower, cut into tiny florets

12 Oz sliced Provolone cheese

Method

1.   Heat 1 Tablespoon of olive oil in a wide pan over med heat till shiny. Put sliced onions to it. & a pinch of salt, stirring till it is coated with oil. Cook, regularly mixing, till the onions become golden brown & caramelized, for 30 to 45 mins. You will need to switch the heat to med-low if you have a boiling burner since you don't want it to burn. Do not mix very much since you want to fully caramelize the bottom.

2.   Put the ready peppers in a big pot when the onions are cooking & cover them with water. Carry to a simmer & simmer for 2 to 3 mins, till just softened. Drain & put on a sheet of paper towel, softly patting a few liquids off; in the 9x13 inch pan, place the peppers, & preheat the oven to 350 deg C.

3.   Heat the leftover 1 Tablespoon of oil over med heat in a wide skillet. Cook your sliced steak till golden brown and the extra fat is drained away. Transfer to a dish.

4.   Put the cauliflower in a big food processor when the beef is cooking & process till "rice-like." Put it right in the skillet that your beef was in & cook over med heat, regularly mixing, till golden brown.

5.   When the beef & caramelized onions are cooked, add them to the skillet & sprinkle them with sea salt. Stir till it's mixed properly.

6.   Stuff each pepper with the combination & put a cheese slice to each seed. (1 oz cheese per pepper half). Bake for around 10 to 15 mins, till the cheese is melted and the peppers are soft. Switch the oven to   the high grill & cook till the cheese becomes golden brown for about 2 to 4 mins.

7.   Enjoy it.

7   Asparagus Stuffed Chicken Breast

Servings: 4 | **Time:** 30 mins | **Difficulty:** Easy

Nutrients per serving: Calories: 241.8kcal | Fat: 9.1g | Carbohydrates: 2.9g | Protein: 34.2g | Fiber: 0.7g

Ingredients

Italian seasoning

1 Lb Chicken Breast

Garlic powder

4 tsp Honey mustard

Sea salt

3 Oz Provolone cheese

1 Tbsp Olive oil

8 Stalks of Asparagus

Method

1.   Oven preheated to 425 degrees.

2.   Cut the chicken breasts in half about the entire way, but leave them intact so that each chicken may fold up. Scatter on the inside of every breast the garlic powder, Italian seasoning & a bit of salt. Drizzle the Italian seasoning on chicken breast outside.

3.   From around inside of every chicken breast, scatter one teaspoon of honey mustard. Lay a piece of provolone, followed by Two asparagus spears, on the top of every chicken. Fold your chicken over &, if needed, protect it with toothpicks.

4.   Warm the oil up over med heat in a big, oven-safe skillet. Put the chicken in & cook for around 2 to 3 mins, till golden brown. On the other hand, flip & repeat.

5.   Cover the skillet with tinfoil & bake till the thermometer inserted into your chicken breast reaches 165 degrees, around 15 mins.

8   Chipotle Healthy Pulled Pork In The Slow Cooker

Servings: 5 | **Time:** 8 hrs 15 mins | **Difficulty**: Easy

Nutrients per serving: Calories: 428 kcal | Fat: 33.7g | Carbohydrates: 3g | Protein: 27g | Fiber: 0.4g

Ingredients

For The Pork And Rub:

½ Med sliced yellow Onion

1/2 Cup Water

1 Tbsp minced fresh garlic

½ Tbsp of Coconut sugar

½ Tbsp of Salt

½ tsp of Chili powder

¼ tsp Cumin powder

¼ Tbsp Adobo sauce from a can of chipotle peppers in adobo sauce

1/6 tsp smoked paprika

Whole wheat for serving

2 Lbs Pork shoulder extra fat removed.

Paleo ranch

Coleslaw mix

Lime Juice

Green tabasco

Method

1.   Put the onion in the bottom of the slow cooker & cut the onion & chop the garlic. One cup of water, pour in.

2.   Mix all of the spices for spice rub in a shallow bowl.

3.   Slice off the pork shoulder with some big, noticeable pieces of fat & after this, rub it all over with spice rub till it is equally coated.

4.   Put the pork on the highest part of the garlic, water & onions, then cook for 6 to 8hrs on high till soft and moist.

5.   If the pork is baked, drain much of the liquid from the slow cooker & put the solids back into the slow cooker.

6.   On a chopping board, move the pork & shred it with two forks.

7.   Move the chopped pork to the slow cooker & combine it with the garlic & onions. Cover till ready to serve

8.   Serve your pulled pork on the bun/lettuce, garnished with ranch coleslaw, mix & a squeeze of the juice of lime & green tabasco.

9   Greek Turkey Meatballs With Feta

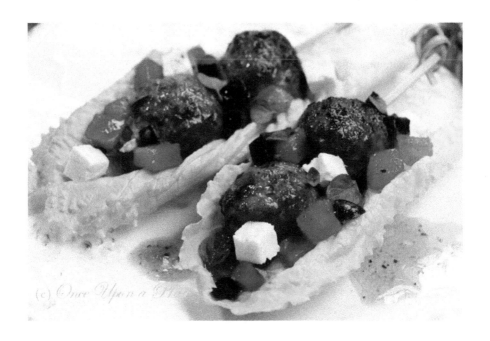

Servings: 4 | **Time:** 30 mins | **Difficulty**: Easy

Nutrients per serving: Calories: 230.4 kcal | Fat: 12.6g | Carbohydrates: 3.2g | Protein: 26.1g | Fiber: 1.5g

Ingredients

2 oz full-fat feta cheese

1 lb lean ground turkey

One big egg whisked

3 tbsp minced fresh parsley

1 tbsp minced fresh mint

2 tbsp coconut flour

1 1/2 tsp ground basil

1 1/2 tsp garlic powder

1 1/2 tsp ground oregano

3/4 tsp ground dill

3/4 tsp cumin

3/4 tsp ground thyme

1/4 tsp ground nutmeg

1/2 tsp salt

1/4 tsp cinnamon

Method

1.   Oven preheated to 400 degrees & use bakery release paper to line a rimmed cookie sheet.

2.   In a big bowl, combine all the ingredients till mixed well. To heap 1 Tablespoon sized balls, use a cookie scoop to put them on the skillet, forming them into a ball. Twenty balls you can have.

3.   Bake till the thermometer reaches 165 degrees F for a moment, around 10 to 13 mins.

4.   Serve & Enjoy.

10   Air Fryer Salmon

Servings: 2 | **Time:** 12 mins | **Difficulty**: Easy

Nutrients per serving: Calories: 183.2 kcal | Fat: 11.6g | Carbohydrates: 0g | Protein: 20g | Fiber: 0g

Ingredients

8 Oz Wild-caught salmon

Sea salt

1 tsp Olive oil

Method

1.   Rub a salmon with the oil of olive & drizzle it with sea salt.

2.   Put in the air fryer's mesh basket & cook at 400 degrees till the temperature reaches 120 degrees F.

3.   Cover & stop for ten min.

11 BBQ Chicken Low Carb Healthy Quesadillas

Servings: 2 | **Time:** 35 mins | **Difficulty:** Easy

Nutrients per serving: Calories: 459 kcal | Fat: 14.4g | Carbohydrates: 19.5g | Protein: 59.2g | Fiber: 7g

Ingredients

1 Cup shredded Chicken breast

2 Cups Liquid Egg whites

Avocado Oil Spray

1/4 cup BBQ sauce of choice + extra for drizzling

2-4 Tbsp Coriander chopped

2/3 cup grated Cheddar cheese

Method

1.   Carry a tiny pot of salted water to a simmer, & cook the chicken breast for around 10-15 mins till it is no longer pink inside.

2.   Preheat the broiler & adjust the oven rack from the top position to the 2nd position. Use Avocado Oil to spray a cookie sheet.

3.   Spray a tiny skillet with Avocado Oil & heat over high heat. Lower the heat when hot, & slowly place a half cup of the white egg in. Cover & cook till just set, around five min, on top of the white egg. Slide the "tortilla" egg on the prepared cookie sheet, & repeat till you have four "tortillas" with the leftover egg whites. Put all the tortillas on the cookie sheet & spray with Avocado Oil on top of them.

4.   Cut the chicken using two forks, then put it in a bowl. Please put it in the BBQ sauce till the chicken is very well covered.

5.   Split the shredded chicken into two of the "tortillas" then stretch out to surround the "tortilla." Split on top of the chicken, the cheese & Coriander, & spray with avocado oil. Cover with the extra tortillas, the un- cooked egg white side down. With Avocado Oil, brush the tops of the quesadillas.

6.   Put the quesadillas underneath the broiler & broil for around fifteen min, till slightly crisp as well as the egg whites start to bubble.

12 Chocolate Coffee Rubbed Steak With Coconut

Servings: 2 | **Time:** 20 mins | **Difficulty:** Easy

Nutrients per serving: Calories: 286 kcal | Fat: 19g | Carbohydrates: 5g | Protein: 24g | Fiber: 1g

Ingredients

1/4 tsp Salt

1 tsp ground coffee

1/4 tsp Garlic powder

1/2 tsp Chili powder

1/4 tsp Onion powder

1/2 tsp smoked paprika

1 tsp cocoa powder, Unsweetened

1/8 tsp Cinnamon

1 tsp sugar of coconut

Pepper Pinch

2 Tbsp coconut flakes, Unsweetened

1/2 Lb Strip steak, New York

Method

1.   Combine the ingredients of the rub in a med bowl & set aside.

2.   Cut the steak off some big, noticeable chunks of fat & cover it with the rub. Get in there for good to ensure that the steak is properly covered.

3.   Cover your steak & let it stay in the fridge for at least one hour, ideally longer to incorporate the flavor.

4.   Spray with cooking spray on a grill skillet (or normal pan) & preheat over high heat. Oven preheated to 400 degrees as well.

5.   Cook the steak, around 1-2 mins per side, till pleasant & seared on either side.

6.   Switch the heat down to med and continue cooking till the appropriate amount of done-ness is met

7.   Move to a plate after the steak is cooked & cover this with tinfoil to sit for 5-7 mins.

8.   Toast the coconut flakes on a tiny, bakery release paper lined cookie tray whereas the steak is resting. See carefully as it requires just 2 min for them to get soft & golden.

9.   Enjoy your steak garnished with a flake of coconut.

13 Pistachio Crusted Chicken With Coriander Yogurt Sauce

Servings: 2 | **Time:** 30 mins | **Difficulty:** Easy

Nutrients per serving: Calories: 409 kcal | Fat: 11g | Carbohydrates: 21g | Protein: 51g | Fiber: 7g

Ingredients

For The Chicken

Salt

1/2 Cup Roasted Pistachios

8 Oz Chicken

One big egg white

For The Cauliflower Rice

4 Cups Cauliflower (cut into bite-sized slices)

1/2 cup Coriander, roughly minced

Salt & pepper

Fresh juice of a lime, to taste

For The Sauce

1/2 tsp Ground cilantro

1/2 cup non-fat Greek yogurt

1/8 tsp Cayenne pepper

Juice of half a lime

Salt Pinch

Method

1.   Oven preheated to 425 degrees & put it on top of a wide cookie sheet with a little cooling rack.

2.   Grind your pistachios & a salt pinch in a tiny food processor till the pistachios are processed but still a little bit chunky. This preserves the crunchy chicken. Place the pistachios into a dish with shallow sides. Put the white egg in a med dish.

3.   Pat your chicken to dry & put in the white egg, shaking off all the surplus. After this, roll about softly, put in the pistachios, so the full chicken is coated, pressing firmly to stick the nuts to a chicken. Put it on the rack & bake for around 12-15 mins till the chicken is no further pink from the inside, & the outside becomes golden brown & crunchy.

4.   Put the cauliflower in a big food processor, whereas the chicken cooks & processes till it appears like rice.

5.   Put in a big bowl & microwave the cauliflower rice till tender, around 3-4 mins. Combine with the Coriander & sprinkle to taste with the salt & new lime juice. Place aside

6.   In a tiny bowl, mix all the sauce ingredients & serve on top of the chicken & rice of cauliflower.

7.   Decorate with it, Coriander.

14   Crock Pot Low Carb Buffalo Chicken Soup

Servings: 4 | **Time:** 4 hrs 10 mins | **Difficulty:** Easy

Nutrients per serving: Calories: 305 kcal | Fat: 26.2g | Carbohydrates: 6.9g | Protein: 11.9g | Fiber: 0.6g

Ingredients

3/4 cup thinly sliced Celery

1/2 Tbsp Ghee

1/4 cup diced Onion

2 cups chicken broth (Low-sodium)

1/2 cup coconut milk (Full fat)

1/4 Cup Hot sauce

1/2 Cup full 30 Ranch dressing

1/2 tsp Sea salt

1/2 Lb Chicken thighs

1/4 tsp Paprika

sliced Green Onion for garnish

1 Tbsp Tapioca starch

Method

1.   Warm the ghee on med-high heat in a wide bowl. Put in the celery & onion, then cook for around 3-4 mins before they start to soften & brown. Put into the 7-quart crockpot.

2.   Cover the chicken with all the leftover ingredients & stir till mixed— Nestle your chicken into a liquid, on HIGH, cover & cook for three hrs.

3.   Stir together the tapioca starch & 2 teaspoons of the liquid of cooking in a med bowl till smooth. Mix it back into the crockpot to ensure that it's smooth & blended—Cook for 1 to 2 more hours, or till the soup hardens a bit.

4.   Remove & chop the chicken from your crockpot. Through the crockpot, mix it back.

5.   Serve it with onion

15   Cauliflower Fried Rice

Servings: 2 | **Time**: 20 mins | **Difficulty**: Easy

Nutrients per serving: Calories: 236 kcal | Fat: 11.4g | Carbohydrates: 24.5g | Protein: 11.8g | Fiber: 6.1g

Ingredients

2 Slices smoked bacon (Thick-cut)

3/4 cup diced Onion

4 Cups Cauliflower florets

1 Tbsp minced Garlic

1/2 cup sliced Green Onion plus extra for garnish

2 Tbsp Water

1 Egg

2 1/2 Tbsp Coconut aminos

Salt and pepper to taste

1/2 Tbsp sesame oil (Cold-pressed)

Sesame seeds for garnish

Method

1.   On med heat, heat a broad wok & cook the bacon till brown & crispy golden, turning once. Remove to a lined paper-towel plate & pat the extra fat off. Set that bacon fat in the skillet aside.

2.   Put the cauliflower florets in a broad food processor as the bacon cooks, and pulsate till rice-like. Place aside

3.   3. Lower the heat to med/high when the bacon is cooked & removed from the grill, & put the onions & garlic. Cook till slightly becomes golden brown, for 1 min.

4.   Put the riced cauliflower along with the green onions sliced & cook for around 5 mins, stirring regularly, till the cauliflower becomes golden brown & soft.

5.   Heat a tiny non-stick skillet on med heat as the cauliflower cooks. Mix the water with the egg & put it in the skillet. Use a cap to protect & cook till the egg is ready. Don't scramble around it. Cut it onto a chopping board till cooked & break it into small slices.

6.   Take it from the heat & stir in the cut egg, coconut amino & sesame oil till the cauliflower is fried. Season with salt & pepper. After this, crumble & whisk in the fried bacon till fairly combined.

7.   Decorate with additional sesame & onion seeds.

16   Coconut Chicken Curry

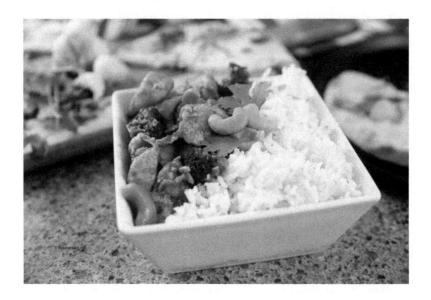

Servings: 6 | **Time**: 40 mins | **Difficulty**: Easy

Nutrients per serving: Calories: 660 kcal | Fat: 60g | Carbohydrates: 7g | Protein: 13g | Fiber: 7g

Ingredients

2 Tbsp divided Coconut oil

1 1/2 lbs chicken thighs (boneless skinless)

One thinly sliced Red pepper

1/2 cup diced Onion

1/2 Tbsp minced fresh garlic

1/2 Tbsp minced fresh ginger,

2 tsp Turmeric

4 tsp yellow curry powder

1 tsp ground cumin

1 tsp Salt

1 tsp Garam masala

1 1/2 Cups Chopped tomatoes

1 Can coconut milk Full fat (14 oz)

1/2 cup minced Coriander

Rice/cauliflower rice for serving

Method

1.   Heat 1 tablespoon of coconut oil on med/high heat in a big, high-sided frying skillet. Include the chicken thighs & cook till seared & golden brown for 1-two min on each side, then move to a tray.

2.   The residual oil is applied as well as the heat is switched to med. Put the onion, red pepper, garlic, curry powder, ginger, garam masala & turmeric , then simmer for around five min, till the vegetables start to soften.

3.   Put the Coriander to the remaining ingredients, & bring to a simmer. After this cover, boil for 3 mins, lower the heat & boil for ten min. Uncover & cook for another 5-ten min till the sauce has thickened significantly.

4.   Take the chicken to a chopping board & chop2 it with two forks, then, together with the Coriander, mix it back into the curry.

5.   Serve with the preferred rice.

17 Low Carb Keto Chicken Stir Fry

Servings: 2 | **Time:** 25 mins | **Difficulty:** Easy

Nutrients per serving: Calories: 238 kcal | Fat: 9.6g | Carbohydrates: 15g | Protein: 27g | Fiber: 4.3g

Ingredients

1 1/2 Tbsp divided Olive oil

1/2 Lb thinly sliced chicken breast (boneless skinless)

1/2 courgette Sliced

One thinly sliced Red pepper

1/4 sliced Onion

1/2 tsp minced fresh ginger

1/2 tsp minced fresh garlic

2 Tbsp soy sauce (reduced sodium)

1/2 Tbsp Rice vinegar

Salt

1/2 tsp Sesame oil

Cauliflower rice for serving

Green onion for garnish

Method

1.   In a wide, elevated side skillet or wok, heat one tablespoon of oil over med/high heat. Cook the chicken for around 5-6 mins, till the center is golden brown & no further pink. Move to the skillet.

2.   In the skillet, Put the leftover oil & switch the heat to a med amount. Put all the vegetables into the soy sauce & cook for around 5-8 mins, till the vegetables are brown & soft.

3.   Return to the chicken & the sesame oil, rice vinegar & soy sauce to the skillet & cook for around 30 sec.

4.   Garnish it with green onion & Serve with rice or cauliflower.

18   Cilantro Lime Cauliflower Rice

Servings: 4 | **Time:** 20 mins | **Difficulty**: Easy

Nutrients per serving: Calories: 113.2 kcal | Fat: 7.1g | Carbohydrates: 11.7g | Protein: 3.4g | Fiber: 4.4g

Ingredients

2/3 cup diced Onion

2 Tbsp Olive oil

One big head of cauliflower, riced

1 Lime juice

1/2 tsp Sea salt

1/2 cup roughly chopped Coriander

Method

1.   In a wide saucepan, heat olive oil to med-high, add onion & cook till soft & slightly browned, around 2-3 mins.

2.   Put the cauliflower rice & cook for around 5-6 mins, constantly stirring, till tender & brown.

3.   Remove & mix in the salt & juice of lime from the heat. Put it all back on the heat & simmer for another 1- 2 mins till a little bit of rice dries out.

4.   Change the salt & lime to taste.

19   Dairy-Free Paleo Casserole With Chicken

Servings: 4 | **Time**: 1 hr 15 mins | **Difficulty:** Easy

Nutrients per serving: Calories: 321 kcal | Fat: 19.8g | Carbohydrates: 13.9g | Protein: 25.2g | Fiber: 4g

Ingredients

The Casserole:

1 Tbsp plus

1 tsp divided Olive oil

1 Lb Lean Ground turkey

1/2 cup diced onion

Pepper

1/4 cup plus 2 Tbsp Tomato paste

One big sliced courgette 1/4 thick 1 tsp minced Garlic

1/2 tsp Salt

1/8 tsp Cardamom powder

1/8 tsp Oregano flakes

1/4 tsp Cumin powder

1/4 tsp Chili powder

1/2 tsp minced Fresh Tarragon plus extra for garnish

1 big thinly sliced tomato

1 cup diced orange bell pepper

For The Sauce:

1 1/2 Tbsp Olive oil

1 Tbsp plus

1 tsp Coconut flour

1 Tbsp plus

1 tsp Almond meal

1 cup Almond milk Unsweetened

Salt & pepper

Method

1.　　oven preheated to 350 degrees & spray the olive oil with an 8x8 inch skillet. Place aside

2.　　Heat 1 Tablespoon of olive oil on med heat in a big saucepan.

3.　　3. Put the turkey & roast till it's no further pink, & the outside is soft & brown. Put the minced tomato paste & onion, then sprinkle with salt.

4.　　Put the sliced courgette and toss with the leftover tsp of olive oil & garlic in a wide bowl. Stir together the cumin, salt, cardamom, chili powder & oregano in a different, shallow bowl. Put & throw in the courgette, ensuring that the spices are uniformly covered.

5.   Scatter the courgette on the bottom of the prepared skillet and scatter the fresh tarragon on the rest of the skillet.

6.   On top of the courgette, scoop the turkey combination & push back so the turkey is soft & wrapped. Place the sliced tomato with an even layer on the turkey top. Finish by splashing the sliced bell pepper uniformly over the surface of the tomato.

7.   Cover and bake the casserole for 15 minutes.

8.   Create the sauce as the casserole bakes by boiling the olive oil over medium/high heat in a wide skillet.

9.   Put flour of coconut & almond meal, then simmer till the flour begins to soak into the oil & give a dark brown color for around 1 min. Think of black peanut butter.

10.   Put in the milk of almond, put it to a boil & whisk continuously. Decrease the heat to mild until boiling so that the sauce remains at a steady low simmer. To make sure it does not smoke, stir regularly.

11.   Cook for around 10-11 mins, till the sauce starts to thicken. With salt & pepper, season.

12.   Place the sauce uniformly till the casserole is cooked & roast, exposed, for another 45 mins.

13.   Let sit for 10 mins; after this slice, Put extra tarragon & enjoy it.

20   Chicken Pesto Spaghetti Squash

Servings: 2 | **Time:** 1 hr 15 mins | **Difficulty**: Easy

Nutrients per serving: Calories: 515 kcal | Fat: 37g | Carbohydrates: 19g | Protein: 31g | Fiber: 4.6g

Ingredients

1 Med spaghetti squash

1 Tbsp divided Oil

8 Oz cubed chicken breast, Boneless & skinless

Salt

Onion powder

Garlic powder

The Pesto:

2 cups lightly packed Basil (32g)

 6 Tbsp Pine nuts

1 tsp minced fresh garlic

1 Tbsp fresh lemon juice

2 Tbsp Olive oil

1/2 tsp Salt

Method

1.   Heat the oven to 400 degrees & use aluminum foil to cover a rimmed cookie sheet.

2.   Break the half-length spaghetti squash carefully & scoop out all the seeds. With 1/2 Tablespoon of oil, massage the inside & season with salt. Put on the cookie sheet, cut-side-down, & bake till the fork is soft, approximately 45 minutes to 1 hour. Additionally, on a small cookie sheet, scatter the pine nuts & bake till about golden brown, around 5-10 mins.

3.   Heat another 1/2 Tablespoon of oil in a wide pan over low heat until the squash is finished. Sprinkle garlic powder, onion powder & salt on the chicken cubes & simmer for around five min, till golden brown.

Make the Pesto

1.   In a Tiny food processor, place the pine nuts & pulse till broken. Put in all the leftover ingredients, excluding the oil, then scrape the sides if required when mixed.

2.   With the food processor going, once well mixed, stream in the liquid.

3.   Split the squash into Two bowls & combine each squash with 1/2 of the pesto. If needed, finish with chicken & extra sliced Basil. Sprinkle with salt to taste.

21   Keto Mexican Cauliflower Rice

Servings: 4 | **Time:** 15 mins | **Difficulty:** Easy

Nutrients per serving: Calories: 109.2 kcal | Fat: 7.2g | Carbohydrates: 10.5g | Protein: 3.5g | Fiber: 4.4g

Ingredients

2 Tbsp Olive oil

2 Lbs cauliflower cut into florets

2 tsp Fajita seasoning

1/4-1/2 tsp Salt

3/4 Cup Salsa of your choice

1/2 cup diced Coriander

Fresh lime juice

Method

1.   In a big food processor, put the cauliflower & pulse till you prefer rice.

2.   Heat oil over med-high heat in a wide skillet. Put the rice & simmer till golden brown, stirring often. Usually 5-6 mins

3.   Put seasoning & salt to the fajita and cook for 1 minute.

4.   Put the salsa & simmer for around 3-4 mins, till the rice starts to dry up. Mix in the Coriander & enjoy it.

22 Keto Creamed Spinach

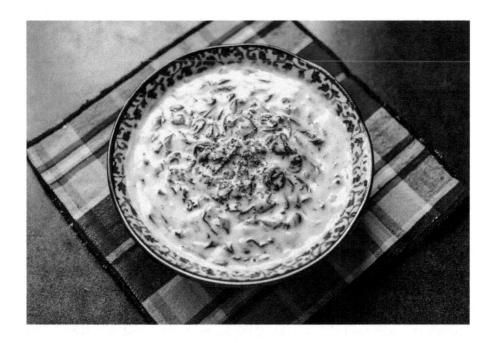

Servings: 4 | **Time**: 10 mins | **Difficulty**: Easy

Nutrients per serving: Calories: 203.2 kcal | Fat: 18.5g | Carbohydrates: 7.4g | Protein: 0g | Fiber: 2.4g

Ingredients

1 Lb Baby spinach

2 tsp Olive oil

2 Tbsp Butter

2 tsp minced Garlic

2/3 cup diced Onion

4 Oz cream cheese Full fat

1/2 cup almond milk Unsweetened

1/2 tsp Salt

1/2 tsp Nutmeg

Method

1.   Heat oil over med heat in a big skillet. Cook your spinach till it is nice & wilted; after this, transfer it to a colander to rinse it.

2.   On a med boil, heat the butter. Put the onion & garlic, then roast for around 3 mins, till golden brown.

3.   Put the almond milk, cream cheese, nutmeg & salt, then mix till the creamy cheese is melted & smooth. Cook for 2-3 mins, constantly stirring, till mildly thickened.

4.   Squeeze out enough water as needed from the spinach & then mix it till well covered in the skillet.

23   No Bean Low Carb Keto Turkey Chili

Servings: 6 | **Time**: 50 mins | **Difficulty:** Easy

Nutrients per serving: Calories: 195.6 kcal | Fat: 10.1g | Carbohydrates: 7.1g | Protein: 20.6g | Fiber: 2g

Ingredients

1 1/2 Tbsp divided Olive oil

1/2 cup diced Onion

One big diced red pepper

1/2 cup thinly sliced Celery

1 Tbsp minced fresh garlic

4 tsp Chile powder

1.25 Lbs Lean ground turkey

1 Tbsp Paprika

1/4 tsp Cayenne pepper

1 1/2 tsp ground cumin

1 Can Fire-roasted minced tomatoes

1 Can Chopped tomatoes

2 Tbsp Tomato paste

1/2 Cup Water

1 tsp Salt Pepper Pinch

2 Bay leaves

1/4 cup chopped Parsley

Method

1.   Heat 1 Tablespoon of oil over med-high heat in a big saucepan. Put the pepper, onion, garlic & celery, and then simmer for around 3 mins until the onion starts to soften.

2.   To the skillet, put the remainder of the oil as well as the turkey. Cook for approximately 3-4 mins, till the turkey, starts to brown. Drain some of the liquid away.

3.   Put in the spices & cook for around 3-4 mins till the turkey is no further pink & the spices become fragrant.

4.   Put the roasted tomatoes, water, smashed tomatoes, tomato paste, pepper & salt on the burner & mix till well mixed. Now Carry it to a simmer.

5.   Mix in the bay leaves after boiling, lower the heat to med-low, & cover the skillet. Boil for thirty min, sometimes stirring.

6.   Remove the bay leaves & mix in the Parsley till they have simmered.

24 Middle Eastern Keto Slow Cooker Chicken Thighs

Servings: 4 | **Time:** 4 hr 10 mins | **Difficulty:** Easy

Nutrients per serving: Calories: 596 kcal | Fat: 35g | Carbohydrates: 3g | Protein: 63g | Fiber: 1g

Ingredients

2 pounds Chicken Thighs Boneless & Skinless

1 tbsp Za'atar Seasoning

1/3 cup Chicken Broth

2 ounces Goat Cheese

3 tbsp Tahini Paste

One tbsp Fresh Juice of Lemon

1/2 tsp Sea Salt

1/2 Lemon

sliced Fresh Mint for garnish

Method

1.   Break off some of the chicken's big noticeable pieces of fat (optional) & place the thighs in the crockpot's rim. Drizzle seasoning on the zaatar & brush all around the chicken to thoroughly cover it.

2.   Put the goat cheese in a med, microwave-safe bowl & microwave for around 15-30 sec, till the goat cheese only starts to soften. Put all the remaining ingredients & mix in a bowl until the cheese is smooth & broken down.

3.   Place on the chicken to make sure that everything is covered. In the crockpot, bring the two halves of Lemon.

4.   Cover & simmer for 4-5 hours on low heat till the chicken is soft and fried.

5.   Squeeze all the juice out from the lemons into the crockpot once it is cooked. Move the chicken to the bowls, mix the leftover sauce till it's mixed in the crockpot.

6.   Spoon the sauce on the chicken & if needed, top with mint.

25   Dairy-Free Vegan Cauliflower Soup

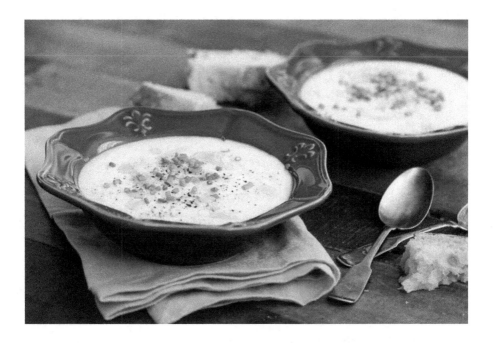

Servings: 6 | **Time: 1** hr 5 mins | **Difficulty**: Easy

Nutrients per serving: Calories: 152 kcal | Fat: 11.7g | Carbohydrates: 10.8g | Protein: 4.8g | Fiber: 4.4g

Ingredients

1 Garlic head

10 Lightly Heaping Cups Cauliflower, cut into florets (one medium head that is 2 lbs 10 oz)

3 Tbsp plus 1 tsp Olive oil

1/2 big roughly chopped Onion

1 1/4 tsp divided Salt

4 Cups Chicken

4 Tbsp cream cheese of Full fat

Method

1.	Oven preheated to 400 degrees.

2.	Break off the top of the head of garlic, reveal the cloves & strip all of the papery skin away. Put the garlic on the highest point of a double layer of the tinfoil, cut-side-up. Put one teaspoon of olive oil on the garlic. To build a tiny package over the garlic, fold the tinfoil from the end, making sure it's securely closed. Put it on a small cookie sheet & bake for around 40-45 mins till the garlic is soft.

3.	Put the cauliflower & the onion in a wide bowl, then toss with three teaspoons of olive oil & 3/4 teaspoon salt. Divide into two cookie sheets equally.

4.	Bake for around 20-25 mins, often stirring, till tender & golden brown.

5.	Put the onion, half Garlic head & cauliflower in a high-powdered processor till it has been roasted. Put 1/2 teaspoon of salt, broth & cream cheese to the leftover 1/2 teaspoon, and combine until smooth and fluffy. If you like, sample the broth, change some salt, and incorporate some garlic.

26   Low Carb Buffalo Chicken Meatballs

Servings: 4 | **Time:** 30 mins | **Difficulty:** Easy

Nutrients per serving: Calories: 378 kcal | Fat: 18g | Carbohydrates: 28.3g | Protein: 30.4g | Fiber: 8.8g

Ingredients

The Zoodles

Eight big courgettes

Salt

For The Cauliflower Alfredo:

3 Cups Water

5 Cups (cut into bite-sized pieces) Cauliflower

3 Cups broth of Vegetable

1 1/2 Tbsp minced Garlic

1 Tbsp Olive oil

1/2 cup roughly chopped onion

Pepper

1/2 tsp Salt

2 Tbsp Milk

The Meatballs:

1 Lb additional Lean Ground chicken

1/2 cup grated Mozzarella cheese

1/4 cup plus 2 Tbsp old fashioned oatmeal (Rolled)

1/4 cup diced Green Onion plus extra for garnish

1 1/2 tsp minced Garlic

1 tsp Salt

1 Tbsp Ranch seasoning

Pepper Pinch

Buffalo chicken sauce

One big egg white

Method

1.   oven preheated to 400 degrees & spray the cooking spray on a baking dish.

2.   On a mandolin, use a 5/7 millimeters julienne blade & slice courgette lengthwise to produce long noodles.

3.   Toss the courgette noodles & let them hang in the strainer on a cup for 20 to 30 mins. A couple of times, mix them around as they strain.

4.   In a big kettle, mix the water and vegetable broth and bring it to a boil. When it is cooked, add the cauliflower and cover it. Cook for around 6-7 minutes until the cauliflower is soft. Remove from the sun, and to stay safe, cover. Don't drain them!

5.   Combine cheese, ground chicken, 1/4 cup of green onion, 1 tsp of salt, 1 1/2 tsp of garlic, ranch powder, oatmeal, pepper & egg whites in a big bowl. Mix, so it's blended equally.

6.   Make the meat into balls & put it on the cookie sheet that has been prepared. Put them in the oven & bake for 10 to 15 mins.

7.   In a med skillet, heat one tablespoon of olive oil & cook the garlic & onion until finely golden brown. In a big food processor/blender, incorporate the cooked garlic & onion.

8.   Move the cauliflower into the food processor with a slotted spoon & put salt, a pepper pinch & cream. Blend & then put 3 to 4 more cooking liquid teaspoons till the required consistency is obtained in the sauce.

9.   Squeeze the courgette noodles out of the excess water and split them between bowls. If required, cover with meatballs, cauliflower sauce & sprinkle with buffalo sauce & additional green onions.

27   Low Carb Pizza Meal Prep Bowls

Servings: 4 | **Time**: 20 mins | **Difficulty:** Easy

Nutrients per serving: Calories: 453.5 kcal | Fat: 29.4g | Carbohydrates: 10.2g | Protein: 36.8g | Fiber: 1.9g

Ingredients

24 uncured Pepperonis Eight slices of Ham

Four slices of Bacon

Two sliced Green Peppers

1 tbsp Italian Seasoning

1 pound Lean Grass-Fed Ground Beef

1/2 tsp Sea Salt

3/4 cup divided Tomato Sauce

1/4 cup sliced Black Olives

3 ounces grated Mozzarella Cheese

Cheese Sauce:

1 cup Roasted Cashews (soaked in water)

2 tbsp Nutritional Yeast

1/3 cup Water

1 tsp Sea Salt

1 tsp Garlic Powder

1/4 tsp Stone Ground Mustard

1/2 tsp Onion Powder

Black Pepper pinch

Method

1.   Oven preheated to 185 °c & use bakery release paper to line a baking sheet. Put the pepperonis & ham out and bake for around 5-10 mins, till lightly crisp. Monitor carefully as before the pepperoni; the ham would most definitely be done.

2.   Fry the bacon till golden brown & on each side in a wide frying pan on med heat, switching to a towel- lined plate & extracting the excess oil once cooked.

3.   Into the skillet, Put the peppers & mushrooms with the remaining bacon fat & fry, constantly stirring, till golden brown & soft, around ten min.

4.   Heat a separate big frying pan on med-high as the vegetable fry, then fry the beef, breaking it as it cooks, till it's no further pink from inside, around 10 mins. Drain the extra fat away.

5.   Stir in the beef with Italian seasoning & salt till well combined. Then put ½ cup tomato sauce & stir.

6.   Divide the pepperoni, ham, vegetables, bacon, olives & meat. Divide per bowl (1 Tablespoon each) with the remaining tomato sauce. Eventually, split the shredded cheese & cover every bowl, then refrigerate till ready to serve! The bowls could last in the refrigerator for 3 to 5 days.

7.   Reveal & microwave for around one minute before ready to eat, or when the cheese melt. Mix & enjoy it.

To make Paleo cheese sauce

1.   Put all the ingredients & blend in a Tiny food processor, preventing scraping down the sides till smooth.

2.   Store in a small separate meal prepared jars.

28   Turkey Meatballs With Basil Black Walnut Pesto Cream

Servings: 4 | **Time:** 30 mins | **Difficulty**: Easy

Nutrients per serving: Calories: 458 kcal | Fat: 34.6g | Carbohydrates: 11.1g | Protein: 26.4g | Fiber: 3.9g

Ingredients

The Meatballs:

1 Egg

1 Lb Lean ground turkey

1/4 cup sliced Fresh Basil plus extra for garnish

2 tsp minced fresh garlic

2 tsp Italian seasoning

1 tsp packed Lemon zest

4 tsp Coconut flour

1/2 tsp Sea salt

1/2 cup chicken broth Reduced sodium

Four small courgettes

For The Sauce:

2 1/4 cups very tightly packed Fresh Basil (35g)

1/3 Cup Black Walnuts, Hammons

2 tsp Lemon zest

2 Tbsp Fresh juice of Lemon

1 tsp minced fresh garlic

2 tbsp additional Virgin Olive oil

3/4 tsp Sea salt

6 Tbsp coconut milk Full fat

6 Tbsp chicken broth Reduced sodium

Method

1.   Mix all the meatball components with the coconut flour in a wide bowl till it's combined. Place the coconut flour in & mix till it's combined. Form into 20 slightly heaping balls.

2.   Heat a big, non-stick skillet on med-high heat. Cook the meatballs along both sides till golden brown - around 1 min per side. Stir in the broth of the chicken, decrease the heat to med/low & cover. Cook for around 8-11 mins, stirring regularly, till the meatballs are cooked as well as the broth has been absorbed.

3.   Put the black walnuts into a Tiny food processor as the meatballs cook, & pulse till broken down. Put all the leftover ingredients & pulse to the olive oil till it is broken down & mixed.

4.   With the food processor going, when well combined, stream in the olive oil

5.　　　Mix the milk of coconut & chicken broth in a big frying pan over med/high heat. Just get it to a simmer.

6.　　　Mix in all the pesto till just mixed & cook for 1 min after boiling, mixing continuously. Then lower the heat to med/low, then boil till the sauce starts to thicken, for 2 to 3 mins.

7.　　　On med-high heat, heat a dry frying pan & cook the courgette noodles till they are only softened around 3- 4 mins. Transfer to a sheet of paper towel & the remaining moisture is gently squeezed out—split　　　b/w four bowls.

8.　　　Mix the meatballs into the sauce & serve with fresh Basil and a squeeze of Lemon, if needed, over the zoodles.

29   Chicken Zoodle Soup

Servings: 22 | **Time:** 8 hrs 20 mins | **Difficulty:** Easy

Nutrients per serving: Calories: 344 kcal | Fat: 20.4g | Carbohydrates: 11.9g | Protein: 26.7g | Fiber: 3.3g

Ingredients

3 Med Carrots

1 Pasture raised stewing hen

Four Celery Stalks

One big onion

Six leaves of Bay

Two full bundles of Parsley, covered & tied with twine full Peppercorns

2 Boxes (not sodium-reduced) chicken broth Whole Star anise seed

courgettes Salt

Method

1.   Put the chicken in the big stockpot

2.   Break each carrot & celery stalk into three big pieces & put them on the chicken's highest point.

3.   Break the onion into big pieces & put the carrots & celery on top.

4.   On top of the herbs, place the packed Parsley & bay leaves.

5. Fill two black peppercorn steel diffusers & put them in the stockpot.

6. Repeat this, in a different diffuser, along with the star anise seed.

7. In the stockpot, place a chicken broth box over the top of it.

8. Till all the components are covered, fill the remainder of the pot with water.

9. Carry the pot to a simmer on high heat, after the switch to med & cover & cook all day long.

10. Remove the vegetables & put them aside till the supply is through simmering. Cut the chicken; it will all fall off the bone & put the fat & any little floaty parts off its top of the stock on the plate & skim.

11. Remove extra fat off the chicken, chop & set aside

12. Depending on the 'chicken flavor you want, taste the stock, and see if it needs some extra salt or any more chicken broth.

13. Using a paper towel, gently push out any extra moisture from the zoodles & then split them   b/w bowls. Stock the spoon on top & incorporate shredded chicken.

30   Mediterranean Egg Muffins With Ham

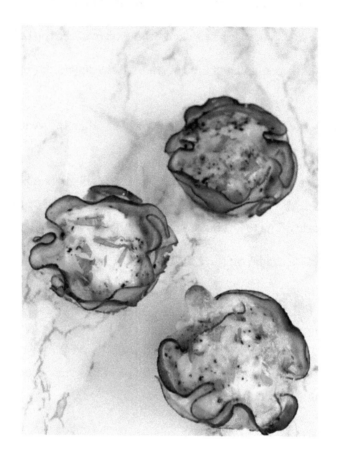

Servings: 6 | **Time:** 25 mins | **Difficulty:** Easy

Nutrients per serving: Calories: 109 kcal | Fat: 6.7g | Carbohydrates: 1.8g | Protein: 9.3g | Fiber: 1.8g

Ingredients

Nine slices deli ham

1/3 cup minced fresh spinach

1/4 cup crumbled Feta cheese

Five big eggs

Salt Pinch

Pepper pinch

Fresh Basil for garnish

1 1/2 Tbsps Pesto sauce

1/2 cup roasted & sliced red pepper (Canned) plus extra for garnish

Method

1.   Oven preheated to 400 degrees. GENEROUSLY brush with cooking spray on a baking tray.

2.   Line every muffin tin with 1 & a half pieces of ham, ensuring that you do not leave gaps to explode out.

3.   On the bottom of each muffin tin, put a tiny bit of roasted red pepper.

4.   On top of every red pepper, put one tablespoon of chopped spinach.

5.   With a heaping 1/2 Tablespoon of crumbled feta cheese, round off the pepper & spinach.

6.   Whisk the eggs along with salt & pepper in a med dish. Divide the mixture of eggs equally between the Six muffin tins.

7.   Bake till the eggs become puffy & sound ready, for 15-17 mins.

8.   Remove the muffin tin from each cup & garnish with 1/4 tsp of pesto sauce, extra red pepper slices & fresh basil.

31   Steak and Shrimp Surf

Servings: 2 | **Time:** 50 mins | **Difficulty:** Easy

Nutrients per serving: Calories: 566 kcal | Fat: 38g | Carbohydrates: 10g | Protein: 41.5g | Fiber: 3g

Ingredients

Filet Mignon:

8 ounces filet mignon

salt & pepper

1 tbsp olive oil

1 cup Monterey Jack cheese

4 ounces softened Philadelphia cream cheese

8 ounces thawed & squeezed dry, frozen spinach

1 tbsp butter

13.75 ounces can quarter artichoke hearts

1/4 cup minced onion

1 tsp minced garlic

1/4 tsp white pepper

1 tsp red wine vinegar

Shrimp Scampi:

Six med shrimp (remove the shell)

salt & pepper

1 tsp minced garlic

2 tsp olive oil

1 tbsp white wine

2 tbsp butter

1 tsp juice of Lemon

1 tbsp minced parsley

Steamed asparagus (prepare in advance, steam before serving)

6 ounces trimmed asparagus

salt & pepper

1 tbsp water

Method

1.   On med heat, put a non-stick plate. When it is hot, Put the onion, garlic &   butter,   cook till tender.   Place the leftover ingredients & mix till the cheeses have melted & cooked through the spinach artichoke sauce. Thin it with water, if you wish. Change the salt & pepper seasonings. Refrigerate until it is cold. It can be completed some days in advance. Heat & stir. Makes 3 cups per serving with 1/2 cup.

2.   Trim asparagus by chopping 1 inch from the bottom and using a vegetable peeler to peel the last Three inches. Bend one spear if the asparagus is small, and it may crack if it is tender. Use it to slice the thickness of the remaining asparagus. Put the asparagus with one tablespoon water in a secure microwave dish & cover with clinging film.

3.   Have the sliced and ready ingredients for its shrimp scampi. Drain a shrimp on a towel, then add salt & pepper on the plate & season.

4.   In a secure microwave dish, place the Spinach artichoke dip & prepare to reheat (or in a small pot on the stove with 1 tbsp of water to reheat on medium-low). Take the asparagus from the refrigerator & prepare it for cooking.

5.   At least 20 to 30 mins before serving, remove the steaks from the fridge. Rub with around one teaspoon of oil on the outer surface, then sprinkle with salt & pepper liberally.

6.   Put a skillet with a hard bottom over the med fire. Place the remaining Two teaspoons of oil when heated, then swirl the skillet to cover the top. Place the steaks as the oil shimmers & do not move for 4 mins. Work a spatula under steaks softly & turn for the next 4 mins to cook. Based on the hardness of the steaks & how cold they become.

7.   Remove your steaks & cover them lightly with foil to settle on a tray.

8.   On med heat, put a non-stick pan. Put the olive oil & tilt when heated to cover the bottom of the plate. Once the oil shimmers, Put the shrimp. Cook the shrimp around 1/2 way up till opaque. Turn over the shrimp & cook for an extra 1 1/2-2 mins.

9.   Remove the shrimp from the bowl, lower the heat, then add the butter & the garlic—1 min to cook. Put the wine and the lemon juice, then simmer till the smell of alcohol in the wine burns away. Take it from the heat & bring the shrimp into the plate, mix in the Parsley & cover loosely with foil.

10.   For 1/2-2 minutes, steam the asparagus. Uh, drain.

11.   Split the steak, shrimp & asparagus into two bowls. Every spinach artichoke dip measures 1/2 cup, saving the remainder for another day. Spoon garlic butter on the asparagus & steak. Now enjoy it.

32   Keto Chicken Marinade

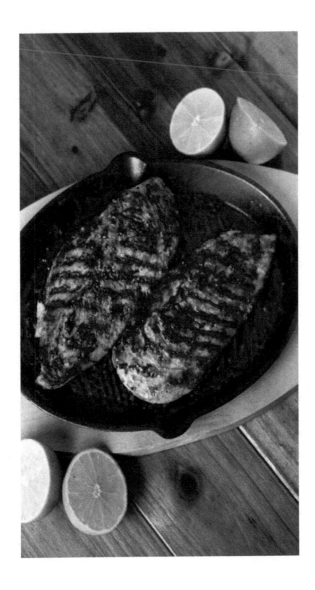

Servings: 1 | **Time:** 5 mins | **Difficulty:** Easy

Nutrients per serving: Calories: 253 kcal | Fat: 27.5g | Carbohydrates: 1.5g | Protein: 1.5g| Fiber: 0.5g

Ingredients

1 lb Chicken breast

2 Tbsps Olive oil

6 Tbsps Chicken broth

1 Tbsp Yellow mustard

2 Tbsps of lemon juice

1 Tsp Dried Italian seasoning

1 Tbsp Minced garlic

Sea salt

Method

1.   Add mustard, garlic, chicken broth, olive oil, lemon juice, seasoning, and salt in a bowl and toss well.

2.   Add the chicken to the bowl and mix everything well. Keep it aside for three hours to marinate.

3.   Heat the grill over medium flame for 15 minutes.

4.   Place the chicken over the grill and grill from both sides for 10 minutes.

5.   Serve and enjoy it.

33   Keto Pork Tenderloin with Pistachio Pesto

Servings: 4 | **Time:** 30 mins | **Difficulty:** Difficult

Nutrients per serving: Calories: 486 kcal | Fat: 27.1g | Carbohydrates: 9.7g | Protein: 50.7g | Fiber: 3.5g

Ingredients

1/3 Cup Salted Pistachios

1/2 Cup cilantro

1 1/2 Cups Basil

½ Tsp salt

½ Lemon zest

1 Tbsp lemon juice

3 Tbsps Olive oil

1 Tbsp Water

½ tsp black pepper

Salt to taste

2 lb Pork tenderloin

1 1/2 Tbsp Olive oil

Black pepper to taste

Method

1.   Place pork tenderloin in a bowl and sprinkle salt, olive oil, and pepper and mix well. Set aside for 15 minutes.

2.   Heat olive oil in a skillet over medium flame and add pork pieces.

3.   Cook for 5 minutes from each side.

4.   Transfer the pork to a baking tray and bake in a preheated oven at 400 degrees for 15 minutes.

5.   Blend the pistachios, basil, lemon zest, cilantro, and lemon juice in a blender to get a granular mixture. Slowly pour in water and oil too to get a creamy mixture.

6.   Now, cook zoodles in a skillet over medium flame until they get soft.

7.   Drain and dry the zoodles and set them aside.

8.   Pour pesto sauce over zoodles and mix well.

9.   Top the zoodles with pork cut into slices and sprinkle pistachios and squeeze lemon juice according to taste.

34 Instant Pot Turmeric Chicken and Vegetables

Servings: 2 | **Time:** 10 mins | **Difficulty:** Easy

Nutrients per serving: Calories: 320 kcal | Fat: 17.3g | Carbohydrates: 10.4g | Protein: 28.4g | Fiber: 4.1g

Ingredients

8 oz Chicken breast

2 Tbsps melted Coconut oil

1/2 Cup coconut milk

1 Tsp minced ginger

2 Tsp Tomato paste

1/4 tsp Ground cinnamon

3/4 Tsp Ground turmeric

Pinch of pepper

Cilantro, for garnish

1/4 tsp Salt

1 Cup Brussels sprouts

1 Cup sliced Broccoli

1/2 sliced Red Bell Pepper

Method

1.   Place the instant pot on sauté mode and heat coconut oil in it.

2.   Cook chicken in an instant pot from both sides for five minutes.

3.   Now, mix coconut milk, tomato paste, ginger, turmeric, salt, and pepper in a bowl.

4.   Transfer the milk mixture to an instant pot and mix well.

5.   Stir in Brussels and shift the mode from sautéing to the manual, and put it on high pressure with a lid on the pot for one minute.

6.   Release the pressure and add bell pepper and broccoli and mix well.

7.   Cover the pot and let it cook for 25 minutes.

8.   Sprinkle cilantro and serve.

35 Asian Miso Steak Sheet Pan Dinner

Servings: 4 | **Time:** 25 mins | **Difficulty:** Easy

Nutrients per serving: Calories: 317 kcal | Fat: 18.7g | Carbohydrates: 11.1g | Protein: 38.5g | Fiber: 4g

Ingredients

4 Baby Boy Choy

4 Cups sliced Broccoli

2 Tbsps White miso paste

Sesame seeds as required to garnish

2 Tsps Sesame oil

2 Tsps Olive oil

1 Lb Sirloin Steak

2 Tsps minced ginger

The Miso Butter:

4 Tsps White miso paste 4

 Tsps Garlic ghee

Method

1.   In a bowl, add boy choy, ginger, broccoli, Misco, and oil and mix well.

2.   Transfer the broccoli over a baking tray lined with a parchment sheet.

3.   Bake for eight minutes in a preheated oven at 400 degrees.

4.   After eight minutes, broil the broccoli for few minutes until they are done.

5.   Now, add all the ingredients of miso butter in a bowl and toss well.

6.   Spread the butter mixture over the steak and set aside.

7.   Sauté the steak in a pan over medium flame for two minutes from both sides.

8.   Transfer the steaks to the side of broccoli and let them broil for five minutes.

9.   Again spread butter mixture over the steak and add boy choy to the other side of the pan.

10.   Let them broil for five more minutes.

11.   Spread the butter mixture again over the steaks and drizzle sesame seeds.

12.   Serve and enjoy it.

36   Sheet Pan Za'atar Chicken Thighs

Servings: 4 | **Time:** 10 mins | **Difficulty:** Easy

Nutrients per serving: Calories: 515 kcal | Fat: 35g | Carbohydrates: 13.4g | Protein: 35g | Fiber: 5.5g

Ingredients

1 ½ Lbs chicken thighs

6 Cups diced Cauliflower

1/4 Cup Pistachios

One sliced onion

2 Tbsps chopped mint

Salt to taste

2 1/4 Tbsps Avocado oil

2 Tbsps Zahtar

2 Tsps lemon juice

4 Tsps Tahini

1/4 Cup chopped Cilantro

2 Tsps Dukkah

Method

1.   Lightly roast the pistachios in a preheated oven at 450 degrees for 10 minutes in a baking tray. Place them aside.

2.   Add salt, olive oil, and cauliflower in a bowl and mix well.

3.   Transfer the cauliflower over a baking sheet. Set aside.

4.   Add zahtar and chicken pieces in a bowl.

5.   Drizzle some salt and transfer it to a cauliflower pan.

6.   Bake the chicken and cauliflower in a preheated oven at 450 degrees for 20 minutes.

7.   Mix tahini, olive oil, and lemon juice in a bowl.

8.   Pour the tahini mixture over the baked chicken pieces and bake for another eight minutes.

9.   Then let them broil for five more minutes.

10.   Drizzle lemon juice over the chicken pieces and sprinkle mint, pistachios, cilantro, and Dukkah, and toss well.

11.   Serve and enjoy it.

37   Tomato Grilled Moroccan Chicken with Yogurt Mint Sauce

Servings: 2 | **Time:** 25 mins | **Difficulty:** Easy

Nutrients per serving: Calories: 205 kcal | Fat: 2.4g | Carbohydrates: 13.1g | Protein: 32.4g | Fiber: 2.8g

Ingredients

1/2 Lb Boneless Chicken breast

2 Tbsps Tomato paste

1/2 Tsp minced Garlic One chopped onion

1/4 Tsp Salt

1/2 Tsp paprika

Pinch of pepper

1 Tsp Olive oil

1/4 Tsp Cumin powder

1/8 Tsp Cinnamon

Mint Yogurt Dip

1/2 Tsp minced Garlic

1/2 Cup Greek yogurt

1/4 Tsp Salt

1/4 Cup grated Cucumber

2 Tbsp chopped mint

Pinch of pepper

Method

1.   Whisk salt, paprika, garlic, olive oil, tomato paste, pepper, garlic, cumin, and cinnamon in a bowl.

2.   Mix in chicken pieces. Place the bowl in the fridge overnight to marinate and to get better results.

3.   Thread the chicken and onion over skewer with alternating fashion.

4.   Place the threaded skewers over a preheated grill and from 15 minutes from all the sides.

5.   Whisk the ingredients of dipping sauce and cucumber in a blender and blend to obtain a smooth mixture.

6.   Sprinkle the mint over grilled skewers and serve with dipping sauce.

38 Oven Baked Mahi Mahi with Macadamia Crust

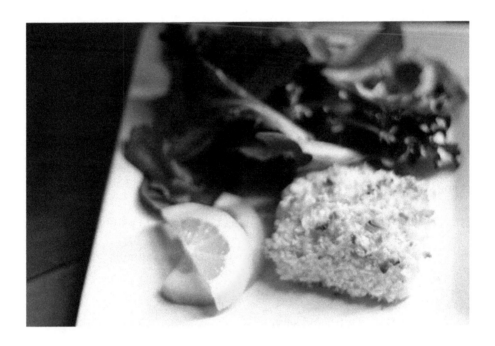

Servings: 2 | **Time:** 20 mins | **Difficulty**: Easy

Nutrients per serving: Calories: 369 kcal | Fat: 27.5g | Carbohydrates: 5.1g | Protein: 28.6g | Fiber: 2.4g

Ingredients

10 oz Mahi Mahi Fillets

1/2 Cup Roasted and chopped Macadamia nuts

1/2 Tbsp Coconut oil

Cilantro as required for garnishing

Salt to taste

Method

1.   Blend nuts in a food processor.

2.   Transfer crushed nuts into a plate.

3.   Drizzle coconut oil over fillets and sprinkle crushed macadamia nuts.

4.   Lightly press the nuts so that they get stick to the fillets. Sprinkle some salt.

5.   Place mahi-mahi fillets in a baking tray lined with parchment paper.

6.   Bake in a preheated oven at 450 degrees for 10 minutes.

7.   Later broil it for five minutes.

8.   Sprinkle cilantro and serve.

39   Spinach Artichoke Greek Yogurt Chicken

Servings: 4 | **Time:** 30 mins | **Difficulty:** Easy

Nutrients per serving: Calories: 320 kcal | Fat: 10.2g | Carbohydrates: 16.9g | Protein: 41.3g | Fiber: 7.1g

Ingredients

For The Chicken:

1/4 Tsp minced Garlic

3 Tbsps Greek yogurt

2 Tbsps artichoke preserving liquid

Four artichoke hearts

½ Tsp salt

1 Lb Chicken breasts

Italian seasoning

½ Tsp black pepper

Spinach as required

The Greek Yogurt Sauce:

1/2 Cup Greek yogurt

1 Tsp chopped Garlic

4 Artichoke hearts

Salt to taste

1/3 Cup blend of grated Parmesan and Romano Cheese

Black pepper to taste

Method

1.   Add yogurt, artichoke liquid, salt, garlic, and pepper in a large mixing bowl. Whisk everything well.

2.   Add chicken in the bowl and toss well to evenly coat the chicken.

3.   Place the bowl in the fridge for three hours to marinate.

4.   Using a sharp knife, make small pockets in chicken pieces and fill them with spinach and place one artichoke heart in each pocket.

5.   Use a toothpick to close the opening.

6.   Drizzle seasoning over the filled chicken pieces.

7.   Place the chicken pieces over a preheated grill and grill for 10 minutes from each side.

8.   Whisk all the ingredients of yogurt sauce in a bowl and blend them in a food processor.

9.   Serve the chicken with yogurt sauce and enjoy it.

40   Indian Salmon Curry Zucchini Noodles with Coconut Milk

Servings: 2 | **Time:** 20 mins | **Difficulty:** Easy

Nutrients per serving: Calories: 408 kcal | Fat: 26g | Carbohydrates: 17.8g | Protein: 27.2g | Fiber: 5g

Ingredients

3/4 Cup coconut milk

Salt to taste

2 tsp Curry paste

8 oz Salmon fillets

The Zucchini Noodles:

Three zucchinis

Salt to taste

Chopped Mint for garnishing

Method

1.   Add salt, coconut milk, and curry paste in a bowl and whisk well. Set aside. The coconut milk sauce is ready.

2.   Place salmon fillets in a baking tray.

3.   Pour the coconut milk sauce over the salmon.

4.   Cover the tray and place in the fridge for three hours.

5.   Drain excess water for zucchini noodles and mix some salt in it.

6.   Place the zucchini noodles aside for 30 minutes with occasional stirring.

7.   Bake salmon fillets in a preheated oven at 450 degrees for 15 minutes.

8.   Add coconut milk sauce in cooked and drained noodles and toss well.

9.   Place baked salmon fillets over the zoodles and sprinkle mint and serve.

41   Low Carb Paleo Zucchini Lasagna

Servings: 8 | **Time:** 1 hr 45 mins | **Difficulty:** Medium

Nutrients per serving: Calories: 367 kcal | Fat: 25.1g | Carbohydrates: 16.7g | Protein: 19.4g | Fiber: 4.2g

Ingredients

The Zucchini Noodles:

1 Tbsp salt

Five zucchinis

For The Meat:

1/2 Lb Pork

1 Cup chopped Onion

1/2 Lb Beef

1 Tbsp chopped Garlic

1 Tsp Dried oregano

1Tbsp Italian seasoning

1/4 Tsp salt

For The Cheese:

2 Cups Raw cashews

1 1/4 Tsp Salt

2 Tbsps lemon juice

1 Tsp Onion powder

Pepper to taste

1/2 Tsp Garlic powder

6 Tbsp Water

Other:

Spice Blend

3/4 Cup Tomato sauce

3/4 Cup Crushed tomatoes

1/2 Cup minced Parsley

1/2 Tbsp minced Garlic

1 Tsp Italian Seasoning

1/2 Tsp Red pepper flakes

1 Tsp Dried parsley

1 Tsp salt

1/4 Tsp Fennel Seed

3/4 Tsp Black pepper

1/4 Tsp Paprika

1/2 Tsp Minced onion

Method

1.   Make thin slices out of zucchini and arrange them on a baking sheet.

2.   Sprinkle salt over the zoodles.

3.   Bake the zoodles in a preheated oven at 350 degrees for 25 minutes.

4.   Add all the items of spice blend in a bowl and mix them well. Divide the mixed spices into two equal portions.

5.   Sprinkle one spices mix portion over the pork pieces and set aside.

6.   Cook sausage, onion, garlic, and beef in a pan over medium flame for ten minutes.

7.   Stir in Italian seasoning, salt, oregano, and black pepper and cook for three minutes.

8.   Transfer the cooked mixture to a bowl and place them aside.

9.   Blend cashews, spices, and lemon juice in a food processor to get a smooth mixture.

10.   Transfer the blended cashew mixture to a bowl and place it aside.

11.   In another bowl, add crushed tomatoes and tomato sauce and whisk well.

Assemble:

1.   In the bowl, first pour a small portion of sauce, followed by the placement of cooked meat, zucchini noodles, cheese mixture, and parsley.

2.   Repeat the same process until everything is used up.

3.   Cover the bowl and bake in a preheated oven for 45 minutes.

4.   Then cook for 15 more minutes while the cover is removed.

5.   Sprinkle parsley over the top and serve.

42   Ham and Asparagus Quiche

Servings: 8 | **Time**: 1 hr 20 mins | **Difficulty**: Easy

Nutrients per serving: Calories: 493 kcal | Fat: 42g | Carbohydrates: 7.5g | Protein: 22.5g | Fiber: 3.8g

Ingredients

One recipe packet of Flaky Pie Crust

1 Cup cubed Ham

8 oz Asparagus

1 Tbsp butter

1 oz chopped onion

¼ Tsp white pepper

2 Cups grated Gruyere cheese

1 Cup heavy cream

Five eggs

¼ Tsp salt

¼ Cup water

Method

1.   Prepare the pie's crust according to the directions given over the packet and chill it until further use.

2. Melt the butter in a pan over medium flame.

3. Sauté asparagus, ham, and onions in the butter with constant stirring until they are done.

4. In the end, add asparagus spears and mix well. Later, separate the spears and set them aside to use them for quiche garnishing.

5. Whisk eggs, salt, pepper, thyme, cream, and water in a mixing bowl.

6. Beat until frothy mixture is obtained.

7. Start making layers of cheese, ham mixture and repeat the process until both are used up over the pie dough in a baking tray.

8. Add custard mixture at the end and spread asparagus spears over the top.

9. Bake in a preheated oven at 375 degrees for 40 minutes.

10. Then, broil for five minutes.

11. Prepare the pie crust per instructions. While the dough chills, move on to the preparation of the quiche ingredients (below).

12. Serve and enjoy it.

43   Crockpot BBQ Chicken

Servings: 2 | **Time**: 3 hrs 35 mins | **Difficulty:** Easy

Nutrients per serving: Calories: 321 kcal | Fat: 16g | Carbohydrates: 5g | Protein: 37g | Fiber: 1g

Ingredients

3 Lbs boneless Chicken breasts

4 oz butter

Sauce Ingredients:

6 oz tomato paste

3 Tbsps cider vinegar

1 Tsp dried thyme

1/3 cup brown sugar

3 Tbsps red wine vinegar

1 Tsp onion powder

1/2 Tsp celery salt

2 Tbsps yellow mustard

1 Tsp garlic powder

1 Tsp salt

1 Tsp liquid smoke

1 Tsp black pepper

1/8 Tsp ground cloves

Method

1.   Whisk all the items of sauce in a bowl.

2.   Place the chicken pieces in the crockpot and pour sauce mixture over
it.

3.   Cover the pot and cook for four hours on high mode.

4.   Shred the chicken and add back to the pot.

5.   Add butter and heat to melt it.

6.   Adjust the taste accordingly.

7.   Serve and enjoy it.

44 Chicken Florentine

Servings: 2 | **Time:** 30 mins | **Difficulty:** Easy

Nutrients per serving: Calories: 560 kcal | Fat: 42.72g | Carbohydrates: 6.63g | Protein: 38g | Fiber: 1.2g

Ingredients

6 oz boneless Chicken breasts

1/2 Cup Heavy cream

1/4 Lb sliced Mushrooms

1/4 Cup White Wine

1/4 Cup Cream cheese

1 Tsp minced Garlic

1 1/2 Tbsp Olive oil

1 Cup Spinach

Method

1.   Rub the chicken with salt, oil, and pepper and set aside for a while.

2.   Heat olive oil in a skillet over medium flame.

3.   Add chicken and cook for 15 minutes from both sides.

4.   Transfer the chicken to the plate and cover it to keep it warm.

5.   Heat olive oil again in the same pan and sauté garlic and mushrooms in it with occasional stirring.

6.   Add wine or chicken broth and mix well.

7.   Stir in spinach and cook for few minutes with stirring until they wilt.

8.   Now create a space in the middle of the pan and add heavy cream and cream cheese in the center and cook to melt them.

9.   Sprinkle pepper and salt and serve.

45   Keto Chinese Pepper Steak

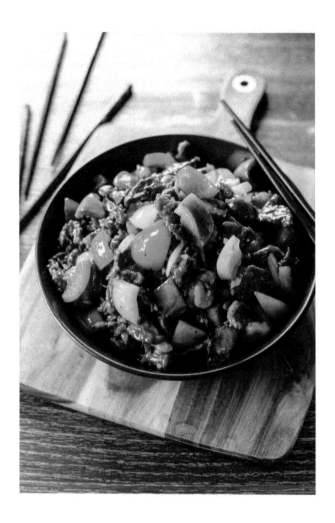

Servings: 3 | **Time:** 25 mins | **Difficulty**: Easy

Nutrients per serving: Calories: 267 kcal | Fat: 16g | Carbohydrates: 5.54g
| Protein: 25.32g | Fiber: 1.3g

Ingredients

12 oz sliced Flank steak

3/4 Red bell pepper

3/4 Green bell pepper

1/4 sliced Onion

1 Tbsp Olive oil

1 Tbsp soy sauce

1 Tsp toasted sesame oil

Method

1. Heat olive oil in a pan over medium flame.

2. Add beef and cook for two minutes without touching it.

3. After two minutes, stir it and cook for two more minutes.

4. Transfer cooked beef pieces into the plate and set aside.

5. Heat olive oil again in the same pan over medium flame.

6. Sauté all the veggies in it. Stir in soy sauce and water and toss well.

7. Cover the pan and let it cook for three minutes.

8. Add beef back to the pan and cook for two minutes.

9. Sprinkle salt, sesame oil, and pepper and serve.

46   Keto Eggplant Lasagna Stacks

Servings: 4 | **Time:** 1 hr | **Difficulty:** Easy

Nutrients per serving: Calories: 255 kcal | Fat: 16g | Carbohydrates: 10g | Protein: 19g | Fiber: 5g

Ingredients

1 1/4 Lbs sliced Eggplant

1 Tsp Salt

1 Egg beaten with

3 Tsps of Water

4 oz sliced Mozzarella cheese

1 Cup Tomato Sauce

1/4 Cup grated Parmesan cheese

1 Tbsp olive oil

Low Carb Keto Breading

1 Cup pork rind panko

1/4 Tsp onion powder

1 Tsp dried oregano

1/2 Cup grated Parmesan cheese

1 Tsp dried basil

1/4 Tsp garlic powder

1/2 Tsp salt

1/4 Tsp ground pepper

Method

1. Slice eggplants and sprinkle salt over them.

2. Place them aside for a while.

3. In a large bowl, beat eggs and set aside.

4. Whisk all the ingredients of breading in a bowl and set aside.

5. Drain and dry eggplants.

6. Dip each of the eggplant slices in the egg mixture and then in breadcrumbs to thoroughly coat the eggplant slices from all the sides.

7. Place the coated eggplant slices on a baking tray.

8. Bake in a preheated oven at 400 degrees for ten minutes.

9. After ten minutes, coat eggplant with tomato sauce and place mozzarella cheese and parmesan cheese over eggplants.

10. Bake again for five minutes to melt the cheese.

11. Serve and enjoy it.

12. Preheat oven to 400 F.

47   Keto Chicken Broccoli Alfredo

Servings: 2 | **Time:** 30 mins | **Difficulty:** Easy

Nutrients per serving: Calories: 534 kcal | Fat: 37g | Carbohydrates: 9.6g | Protein: 42.7g | Fiber: 2.8g

Ingredients

6 oz boneless chicken breasts

1 Cup Broccoli

2 Tbsp Butter

2 Tbsp Water

Black pepper to taste

1/3 Cup Heavy cream

1 Tsp minced Garlic

2 oz grated Parmesan cheese

Salt to taste

1 Cup Cauliflower rice

Chopped parsley for garnish

Method

1.   Rub black pepper and salt over the chicken and set aside for a while.

2.   Melt the butter in a pan over medium flame.

3.   Add the chicken and cook for seven minutes from both sides.

4.   Transfer the cooked chicken to a plate and cover it to keep it warm.

5.   In the same pan, add broccoli and water. Mix and cover the pan and let it steam for three minutes.

6.   Shift the broccoli to the plate with chicken.

7.   Again melt butter in the pan.

8.   Sauté garlic in butter over medium flame.

9.   Stir in heavy cream and cheese and cook while stirring for seven minutes.

10.   Pour in water to bring sauce to the required consistency.

11.   In the end, add pepper and salt and stir well.

12.   Take another pan and melt butter in it over medium flame.

13.   Sauté cauliflower rice and cook for few minutes until cauliflower gets soft.

14.   Sprinkle salt and pepper and toss well.

15.   Serve cauliflower with sauce, chicken, and broccoli, and enjoy it.

48 Vegetarian Keto Lasagna with Mushroom Ragu

Servings: 8 | **Time:** 1 hr 30 mins | **Difficulty:** Easy

Nutrients per serving: Calories: 347 kcal | Fat: 24.64g | Carbohydrates: 11g | Protein: 21.55g | Fiber: 3g

Ingredients

1 ½ Lbs Eggplant

1/2 Tsp dried Basil

1 Lb Mushrooms

1/2 Cup (30 g) Parmesan cheese

3 Tbsps Olive oil

Three sliced Garlic cloves

1 1/2 Cup Marinara Sauce

15 oz Ricotta cheese

1 Egg beaten

3 Cups grated Mozzarella cheese

Eggplant (Preheat oven to 400F)

Method

1.   Sliced the eggplants in eight parts and cut them vertically.

2.   Arrange the eggplants pieces in a baking tray sprayed with oil.

3.   Bake in a preheated oven at 400 degrees for ten minutes from both sides.

4.   Transfer the eggplants to a plate and place them aside.

Mushrooms Ragu: 1.   Roughly chop the mushrooms in a food processor using metal blades.

2.   Heat olive oil in a pan over medium flame.

3.   Sauté garlic in heated oil for one minute.

4.   Stir in chopped mushrooms and cook for few minutes.

5.   Pour in marinara sauce and basil and mix well.

6.   Let the mixture simmer till the point when the desired consistency of the sauce is achieved.

7.   Remove the pan from the flame and set it aside.

Ricotta Cheese: 1. Whisk ricotta cheese with mozzarella and parmesan cheese, and egg. Set aside.

Layer: 1.   Spread sauce in a pan, add eggplant slices, spread ricotta cheese mixture, mushroom ragu, parmesan cheese, and at the end, a layer of mozzarella cheese.

2.   Continue making layers in the same manner.

Bake: 1. Cover the pan with foil and bake in a preheated oven at 375 degrees for 30 minutes.

2.   Uncover the pan and bake for ten more minutes.

3.   Cool the lasagna and slice it to the desired size.

49   Low Carb BBQ Chicken Enchiladas

Servings: 8 | **Time:** 1 hr | **Difficulty:** Easy

Nutrients per serving: Calories: 306 kcal | Fat: 13.55g | Carbohydrates: 18g | Protein: 30g | Fiber: 9g

Ingredients

4 Cups shredded Chicken

1/2 Tsp granulated garlic

3/4 Tsp ground Cumin

2/3 Cup BBQ sauce

2 Tbsps water

1/4 Cup chopped onions

1/4 Tsp white pepper

2 Cups shredded cheddar cheese

1/2 Tsp Pink Salt

8 Tortillas

1 1/4 Cup enchilada sauce

Cilantro for garnish

Method

1.   Whisk BBQ sauce, water, and enchilada sauce in a bowl and set aside.

2.   In another bowl, add chicken, onions, salt, cumin, pepper, and garlic, and toss well.

3.   Add cheese and BBQ enchilada sauce mixture and toss well.

4.   Spread the BBQ sauce mixture in a casserole pan.

5.   Lightly toast the tortillas.

6.   Spread filling over the half section of the tortilla.

7.   Place the tortilla in a casserole pan facing the filling side downwards.

8.   When you are done with all the tortillas, then spread the BQQ sauce and cheese mixture over the casserole.

9.   Cover the pan with foil.

10.   Bake in a preheated oven at 375 degrees for 30 minutes.

11.   Uncover the pan and broil for five minutes.

12.   Sprinkle cilantro and serve.

50 Keto Eggplant Lasagna with Meat Sauce

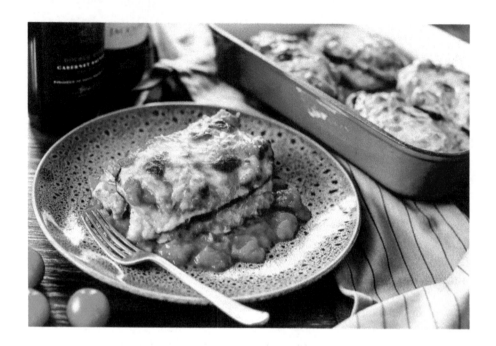

Servings: 8 | **Time:** 1 hr 30 mins | **Difficulty**: Easy

Nutrients per serving: Calories: 410 kcal | Fat: 28.33g | Carbohydrates: 8.85g | Protein: 29.55g | Fiber: 2.4g

Ingredients

1 1/2 Lbs Eggplant

Two chopped Garlic cloves

3 Tbsps Olive oil

1 Lb lean ground beef

3 Cups Mozzarella cheese

1/2 Tsp dried Basil

1 Tsp Roasted Beef Base

1 1/2 Cups Keto Tomato Sauce

1 Egg

15 oz Ricotta cheese

1/2 Cup grated Parmesan cheese

Method

1.   Cut the top and bottom sides of the eggplant. Put the eggplant vertically on the cutting board and make eight pieces out of it.

2.   Arrange the eggplant slices over the cookie sheets sprayed with oil.

3.   Bake in a preheated oven at 400 degrees for ten minutes from both sides.

4.   Transfer the baked eggplant slices into the plate and place it aside.

Meat Sauce:

1.   Sauté garlic in heated olive oil in a saucepan over medium heat for a minute.

2.   Add beef in garlic and cook while breaking it.

3.   Add marinara sauce, basil, and beef base and mix well.

4.   Let it simmer for a few minutes.

5.   When the sauce becomes thick, remove the pan from the flame and set it aside.

6.   The meat sauce is ready. Ricotta Cheese

1.   Add egg and ricotta cheese in a bowl and whisk well.

2.   Add parmesan cheese and mozzarella cheese and mix well again. Set aside.

Layer:

1.   Pour half of the sauce into a lasagna pan.

2.   Place eggplant slices in a pan.

3.   Then pour ricotta cheese sauce followed by spreading of meat sauce.

4.   Repeat the process and make layers until all the items are used up.

Bake (Preheat oven to 375 F):

1.   Cover the pan with butter paper.

2.   Bake in a preheated oven at 375 degrees for 30 minutes while covering the pan with foil.

3.   Uncover the pan and bake for ten more minutes.

4.   Let it cool, and then slice it.

5.   Serve and enjoy it.